HOW TO DRIVE YOUR MAN CRAZY IN BED

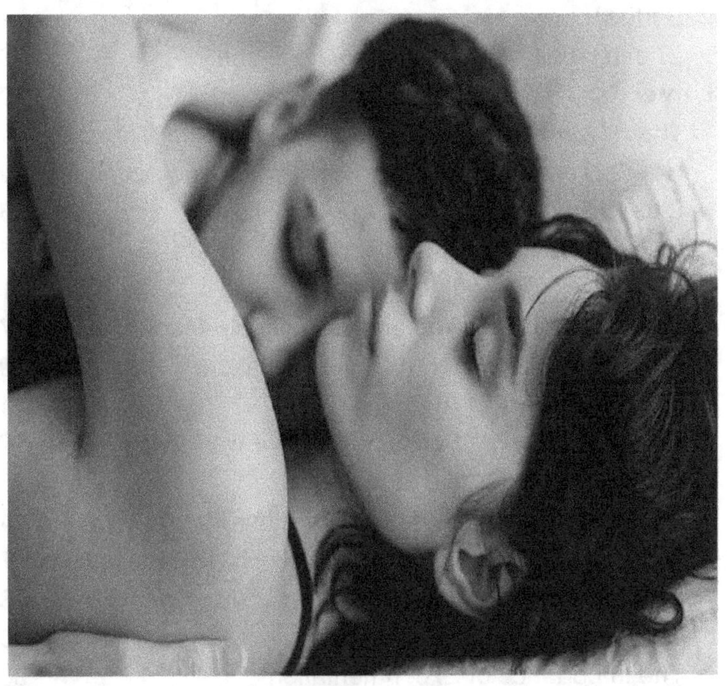

Tease, Ride, and Please him

TABLE OF CONTENTS

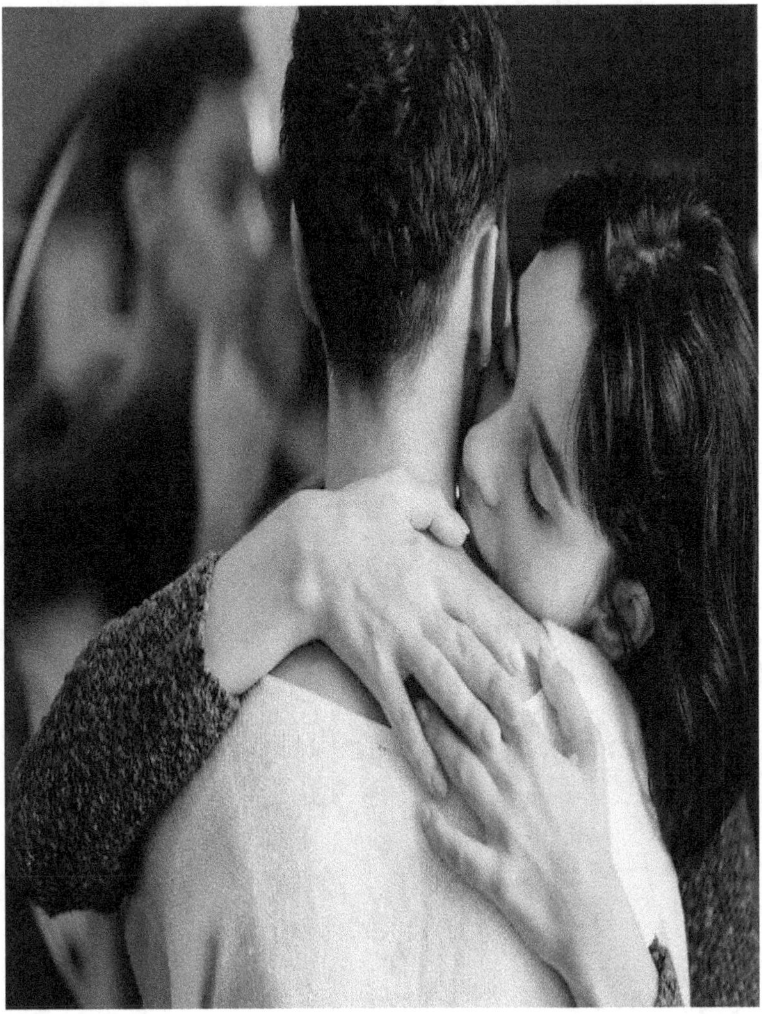

Chapter 1: Introduction

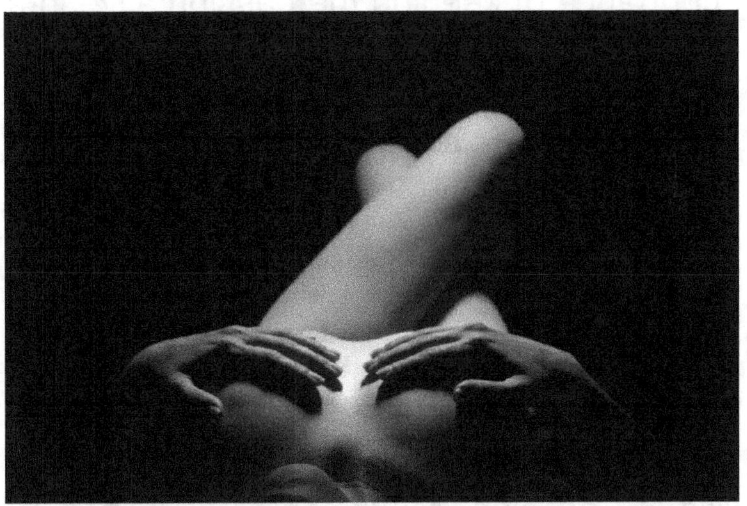

Maintaining a healthy and fulfilling romantic relationship is crucial for our mental and emotional well-being. One of the key factors that contribute to a successful relationship is keeping the passion alive. Passion is what makes a relationship exciting, and it is what keeps us connected to our partners. However, over time, it is common for passion to fade, and relationships can become stale.

In this chapter, we will explore the importance of keeping the passion alive in a relationship, the benefits of being sexually adventurous with your partner, and understanding the male sexual psyche.

The Importance of Keeping the Passion Alive in a Relationship

Passion is what sets romantic relationships apart from platonic ones. It is what makes us feel alive and connected to our partners. Without passion, relationships can become dull, and partners can start to feel disconnected from each other. The importance of keeping the passion alive in a relationship cannot be overstated.

There are several ways to keep the passion alive in a relationship. One of the most important ways is through physical intimacy. Regular physical intimacy, including cuddling, kissing, and sex, can help couples feel closer to each other and strengthen their emotional connection. Other ways to keep the passion alive in a relationship include spending quality time together, engaging in shared hobbies, and communicating openly and honestly.

The Benefits of Being Sexually Adventurous with Your Partner

Sexual intimacy is an essential part of any romantic relationship. Being sexually adventurous with your partner can bring excitement and novelty to your sex life, which can help keep the passion alive in your relationship.

Sexual exploration can also help couples learn more about each other's desires and preferences, which can lead to a deeper emotional connection. Trying new things in the bedroom can also help partners break out of sexual ruts and rekindle the passion in their relationship.

Understanding the Male Sexual Psyche

Understanding the male sexual psyche is an essential aspect of maintaining a healthy and fulfilling romantic relationship. Men and women have different sexual needs and desires, and it is important for partners to understand each other's sexual psychology.

One common misconception about men is that they are only interested in sex for physical pleasure. However, this is not entirely accurate. Men also crave emotional intimacy and connection, and sex is often a way for them to express these feelings. Additionally, men may have different sexual fantasies and desires than women, and it is important for partners to communicate openly and honestly about these topics.

Maintaining a passionate and fulfilling romantic relationship is crucial for our mental and emotional well-being. Keeping the passion alive in a relationship through physical intimacy, shared hobbies, and open communication can help strengthen the emotional connection between partners. Being sexually adventurous with your partner can bring excitement and novelty to your sex life and help partners learn more about each other's desires and preferences. Finally, understanding the male sexual psyche is an essential aspect of maintaining a healthy and fulfilling romantic relationship.

Chapter 2: The Art of Teasing

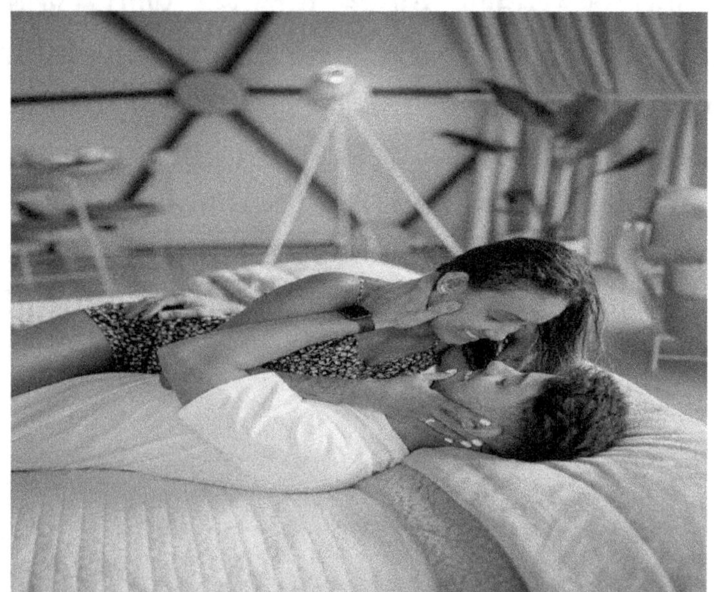

Teasing is an essential part of sexual play and can significantly enhance the experience for both partners. The art of teasing involves creating sexual tension through words and actions, which can increase anticipation and heighten pleasure. In this chapter, we will explore the power of anticipation in building sexual tension, how to tease your partner with words and actions, and different ways to tease your man in bed.

The Power of Anticipation in Building Sexual Tension

Anticipation is a powerful tool in building sexual tension, which is the key to a satisfying sexual experience. Teasing your partner and creating a sense of anticipation can be as pleasurable as the act of sex itself. The anticipation of what is to come can create a heightened sense of desire, making the eventual release all the more satisfying.

When you tease your partner, you are creating a sense of anticipation that builds gradually over time. This slow build-up of sexual tension can create a more intense and satisfying release. Anticipation can be created in a variety of ways, including through teasing words, seductive body language, and tantalizing touches.

How to Tease Your Partner with Words and Actions

Teasing your partner with words and actions can be a powerful way to build sexual tension. Here are some tips on how to do it effectively:

- Use suggestive language: Use suggestive language to build anticipation and create a sense of desire. You can use innuendos, double and other suggestive language to tease your partner and create a sense of anticipation.

- Use your body language: Your body language can be just as powerful as your words. Use eye contact, body positioning, and other nonverbal cues to communicate your desire and create a sense of anticipation.

- Start slow: Teasing is all about building anticipation, so start slow and gradually increase the intensity. Take your time, and enjoy the process.

- Be playful: Teasing should be playful and fun. Don't take it too seriously, and enjoy the moment.

Different Ways to Tease Your Man in Bed

There are many different ways to tease your man in bed. Here are a few ideas to get you started:

- Use your hands: Use your hands to explore your partner's body, but don't give him what he wants right away. Tease him by touching him in all the right places but avoiding his most sensitive areas.

- Use your mouth: Use your mouth to kiss and nibble on your partner's neck, ears, and other erogenous zones. Take your time and enjoy the moment.

- Use props: Use props like blindfolds, feathers, or ice cubes to tease your partner and create a sense of anticipation.

- Use dirty talk: Use dirty talk to build anticipation and communicate your desire. Tell your partner what you want to do to him, but don't give him everything he wants right away.

- Use roleplay: Use roleplay to create a sense of anticipation and add an element of excitement to your sexual play. Dress up in costumes or take on different personas to spice things up.

In conclusion, teasing is an art that can significantly enhance the sexual experience for both partners. By creating a sense of anticipation through words and actions, you can build sexual tension and make the eventual release all the more satisfying. Use these tips and ideas to tease your partner and create a more intense and pleasurable sexual experience.

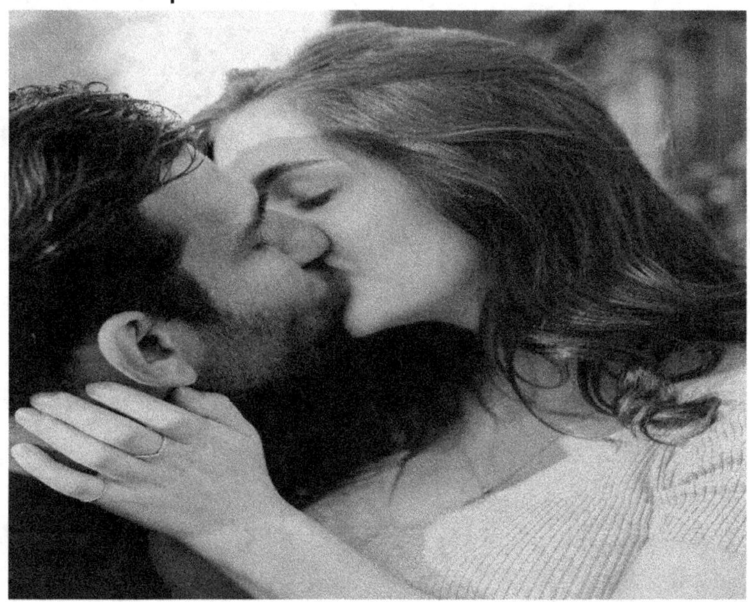

Chapter 3: The Art of Riding

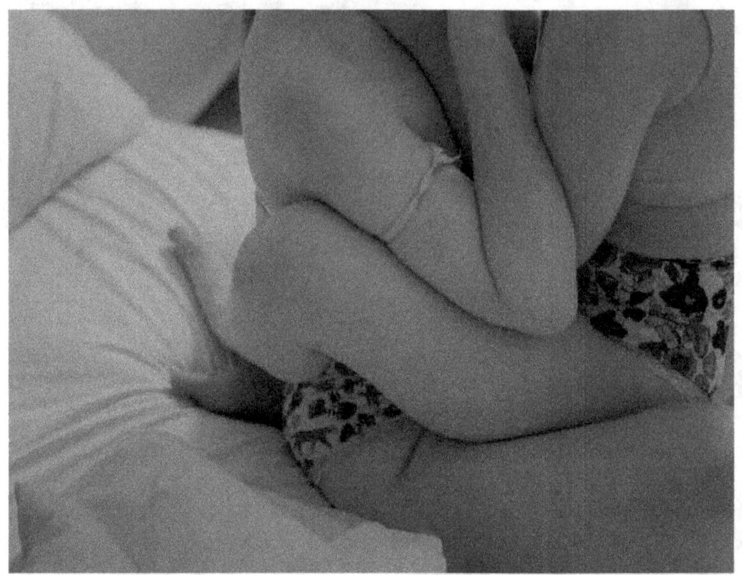

The act of being in control during sexual intercourse can be exhilarating and empowering for both partners. The art of riding, or female superior position, allows women to take the reins and fully explore their sexuality while providing maximum pleasure to their partners. In this chapter, we will discuss the importance of being in control in bed, tips for taking charge and riding your man, and different positions for maximum pleasure.

Understanding the Importance of Being in Control in Bed

The female superior position is not only a great way to take charge and explore your sexuality, but it also provides several benefits for both partners. Firstly, it allows women to control the pace and depth of penetration, making it easier to reach orgasm. Secondly, it allows men to experience new and intense sensations that they may not have felt in other positions. Lastly, it can help create a stronger emotional connection between partners, as it requires trust, communication, and vulnerability.

Tips for Taking Charge and Riding Your Man

1. Get comfortable: Before you begin, make sure you are comfortable and

confident. Take a few deep breaths, relax your body, and focus on the pleasure you want to experience.

2. Communication is key: Let your partner know what you want and what feels good. This can include the speed, depth, and angle of penetration. Don't be afraid to use your voice to guide your partner.

3. Use your hips: The key to a successful ride is to move your hips in a circular or back-and-forth motion. Experiment with different rhythms and see what feels best for you.

4. Incorporate other erogenous zones: Use your hands, lips, and tongue to stimulate your partner's other erogenous zones while riding them. This can include their neck, chest, nipples, and ears.

5. Experiment with different angles: The beauty of the female superior position is that there are several different angles you can try. Experiment with leaning forward or backward, or even sitting upright to find what works best for you.

Different Positions for Maximum Pleasure

1. The classic cowgirl: In this position, the woman straddles her partner and moves up and down, controlling the depth and pace of penetration.

2. Reverse cowgirl: Similar to the classic cowgirl, but the woman faces away from her partner. This position allows for deep penetration and can provide intense G-spot stimulation.

3. The lotus: The lotus position involves the woman sitting on her partner's lap with her legs wrapped around his

waist. This position allows for deep penetration and can create a strong emotional connection.

4. The lap dance: In this position, the woman straddles her partner and moves in a circular motion, similar to a lap dance. This can be a great way to tease and build sexual tension.

The art of riding is a powerful and pleasurable way for women to take control in bed and explore their sexuality. By using communication, experimentation, and different positions, you can create a unique and fulfilling sexual experience for both you and your partner.

Chapter 4: The Art of Pleasing

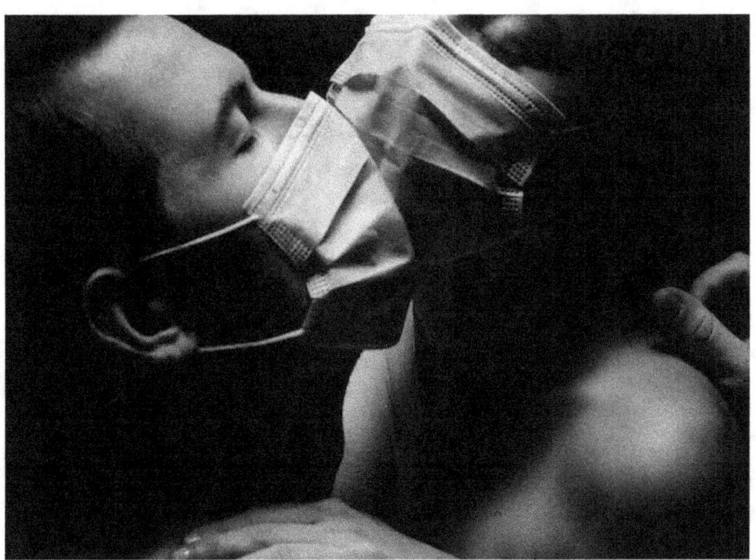

When it comes to sexual intimacy, the focus should always be on mutual pleasure. One of the most important aspects of pleasing your partner is understanding their desires and working to satisfy them. In this chapter, we'll explore the art of pleasing your partner, specifically focusing on techniques for giving oral sex and using your hands to drive your man wild.

The Importance of Focusing on Your Partner's Pleasure

When you're intimate with your partner, it's important to prioritize their pleasure just as much as your own. This means taking the time to explore their body and understanding what feels good for them. Communication is key, so don't be afraid to ask your partner what they like and what they don't like.

Focusing on your partner's pleasure can have a number of benefits for your relationship. It can increase intimacy and strengthen your emotional bond, as well as improve sexual satisfaction for both partners. In fact, research has shown that couples who prioritize their partner's pleasure have higher levels of relationship satisfaction and sexual fulfillment.

Techniques for Giving Oral Sex

Oral sex is a highly personal and intimate act that requires a lot of trust and communication between partners. When performed correctly, it can be incredibly pleasurable for both parties. Here are a few techniques for giving oral sex:

1. Build anticipation: Before diving in, take your time to build anticipation. Kiss and caress your partner's body, and make your way slowly down to their genitals.

2. Use your hands: Incorporating your hands can add extra stimulation and pleasure. Use your hands to stroke, caress, and massage your partner's genitals while you perform oral sex.

3. Pay attention to the clitoris: The clitoris is the most sensitive part of the female genitalia, so it's important to give it extra attention. Use your

tongue and lips to gently stimulate the clitoris, paying attention to your partner's reactions to find the right speed and pressure.

4. Experiment with different techniques: Everyone's preferences are different, so don't be afraid to try different techniques and see what works best for your partner. Some women prefer direct stimulation, while others prefer indirect stimulation.

5. Communicate: As always, communication is key. Ask your partner what feels good and what doesn't, and be open to feedback.

How to Use Your Hands to Drive Your Man Wild

Using your hands during sex can add an extra level of pleasure and intimacy for both partners. Here are a few techniques for using your hands to drive your man wild:

1. Play with the testicles: The testicles are highly sensitive and can provide a lot of pleasure when stimulated. Gently massage and play with them during foreplay and intercourse.

2. Use a firm grip: When giving a hand job, use a firm grip and apply pressure to the base of the penis. Experiment with different speeds and rhythms to find what feels best for your partner.

3. Explore erogenous zones: The male body is full of erogenous zones, so don't be afraid to explore. Kiss and nibble on his neck, ears, and nipples, and use your hands to massage his back, thighs, and buttocks.

4. Incorporate oral sex: Combining oral sex with manual stimulation can be incredibly pleasurable for your partner. Use your mouth to stimulate the head

of the penis while your hand strokes the shaft.

5. Communicate: As always, communication is key. Ask your partner what feels good and what doesn't, and be open to feedback.

The art of pleasing your partner is an important aspect of any sexual relationship. By focusing on your partner's pleasure and exploring different techniques for giving oral sex and using your hands, you can enhance your sexual experiences and create a deeper sense of intimacy with your partner. Remember to communicate with your partner and ask for feedback, and always approach sex with care and consideration.

Chapter 5: Combining Teasing, Riding, and Pleasing

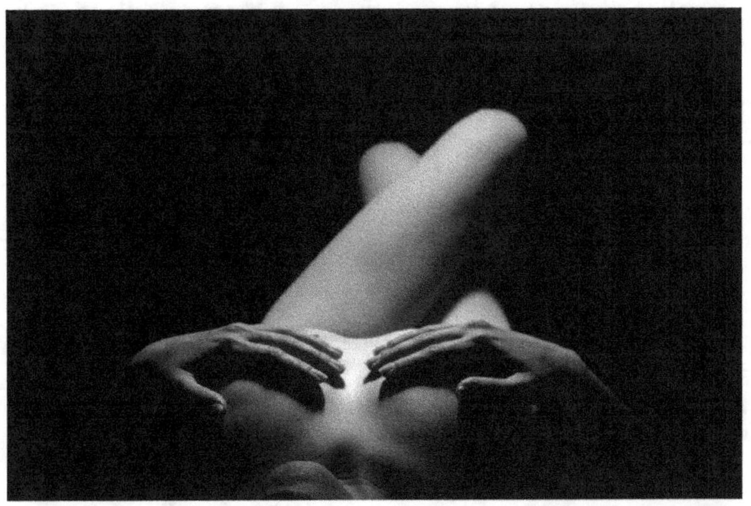

Sexual experiences can vary greatly depending on the techniques and skills employed by partners. Chapter 5 of this guide focuses on bringing together the skills of teasing, riding, and pleasing to create a mind-blowing sexual experience. In addition to this, the chapter also emphasizes the importance of communication and experimentation during sexual encounters.

Bringing All the Skills Together

Teasing, riding, and pleasing are individual skills that can be combined to create a heightened sexual experience. Teasing involves arousing your partner through physical or verbal actions. It could be through kissing, touching, or whispering seductively. Riding, on the other hand, refers to sexual positions where one partner is on top of the other, controlling the pace and depth of penetration. Finally, pleasing involves stimulating your partner's erogenous zones, such as the clitoris or nipples.

When combined, these skills can create a sexual experience that is both intimate and exhilarating. For instance, during foreplay, you could tease your partner by kissing and nibbling their neck while using your hands to stimulate their genitals. As you progress to the main event, you could transition to a riding position, allowing your partner to control the depth and speed of penetration while you continue to tease and please them. This combination of skills can create a more intense orgasmic experience for both partners.

Communication During Sex

Effective communication during sex is crucial for a satisfying experience. Partners should feel comfortable expressing their desires, boundaries, and preferences to each other. This can be done through verbal communication or non-verbal cues such as body language. Communication helps to build trust and intimacy, which can lead to a more fulfilling sexual experience.

During sex, partners should communicate their likes and dislikes, and provide feedback to each other. This can be done through moans, groans, and other vocalizations or by physically guiding your partner's hands or hips. If something is uncomfortable or painful, partners should communicate this to each other to avoid causing harm. Effective communication during sex can lead to a better understanding of each other's bodies, likes, and dislikes, leading to more pleasurable experiences in the future.

The Importance of Experimentation

Sexual experimentation involves trying new things in the bedroom. This could involve trying different sexual positions, incorporating sex toys, or exploring new erogenous zones. Experimentation can help partners discover what they like and dislike, leading to a more fulfilling sexual experience.

When experimenting, partners should take things slow and communicate with each other. It is important to establish boundaries and ensure that both partners are comfortable with the activities being explored. Experimentation should be a fun and exciting experience that brings partners closer together and deepens their connection.

Chapter 5 of this guide emphasizes the importance of combining the skills of teasing, riding, and pleasing for a more intense sexual experience. Effective communication during sex is also crucial for a satisfying experience, as it builds trust and intimacy. Finally, experimentation and trying new things can help partners discover what they like and dislike, leading to a more fulfilling sexual experience. By incorporating these skills and practices, partners can create a sexual experience that is both pleasurable and intimate.

Chapter 6: Tips for Making It Even Better

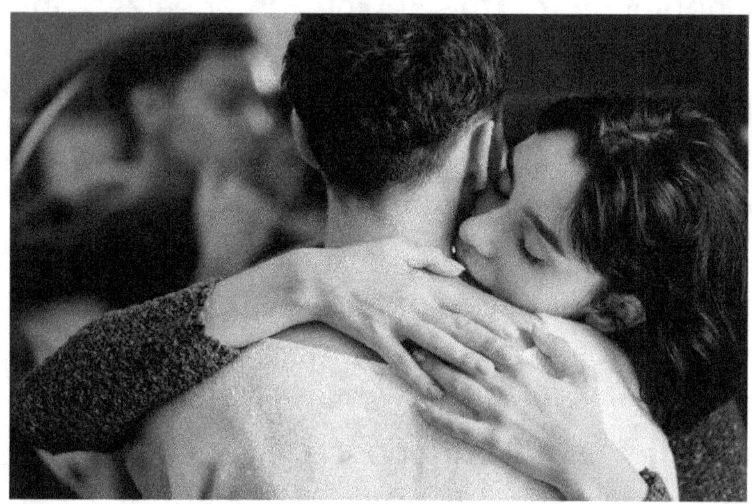

Sexual intimacy is a vital component of any romantic relationship, and it is natural to want to explore new ways to enhance your sexual experience. Incorporating toys and other props into your sex life, exploring role-playing and fantasies, and building trust through open communication are some effective ways to make your sexual relationship even better.

1. **How to incorporate toys and other props into your sex life:**

Using toys and other props during sex can add an element of excitement and variety to your sexual experience. There are various types of toys and props available in the market, such as vibrators, dildos, handcuffs, blindfolds, and massage oils, among others. However, before introducing any toy or prop into your sex life, it is crucial to have an open conversation with your partner and make sure that both parties are comfortable and consenting.

2. **Role-playing and fantasies to explore:**

Role-playing and exploring sexual fantasies can be an excellent way to spice up your sexual relationship. Role-playing allows you to explore different scenarios and act out different roles, which can be exciting and arousing. Some popular role-playing scenarios include doctor-patient, boss-secretary, and teacher-student. Additionally, exploring sexual fantasies can help you identify your desires and communicate them effectively with your partner. However, it is crucial to ensure that both parties are comfortable and consenting before exploring any sexual fantasy or engaging in role-play.

3. **The importance of open communication and building trust in your sexual relationship:**

Open communication and building trust are essential components of a healthy sexual relationship. It is crucial to have open and honest communication with your partner about your likes, dislikes, and boundaries to ensure that both parties feel heard and respected. Additionally, building trust by respecting your partner's boundaries and being responsive to their needs can help create a safe and secure space for sexual exploration.

Incorporating toys and other props into your sex life, exploring role-playing and fantasies, and building trust through open communication are effective ways to make your sexual relationship even better. However, it is crucial to ensure that both parties are comfortable and consenting before exploring any new sexual activity, and maintaining open communication and trust is essential for a healthy sexual relationship.

Chapter 7: Conclusion

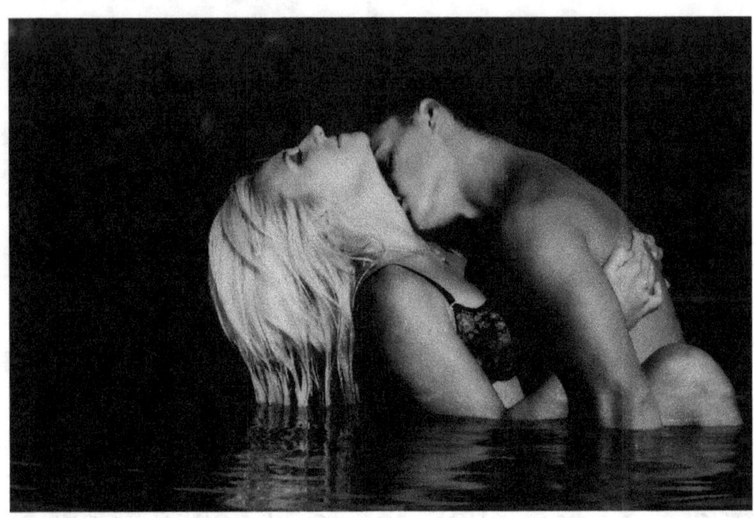

A healthy and satisfying sex life is an important aspect of a successful relationship. Sex is not only a physical act but also an emotional and psychological one. It can bring couples closer together and enhance their intimacy and connection. This chapter discusses the importance of a healthy and satisfying sex life in a relationship, how to continue to explore and experiment in your sexual relationship, and the benefits of a strong sexual connection with your partner.

The Importance of a Healthy and Satisfying Sex Life in a Relationship

Sex is a natural part of human life, and it can be a powerful force that brings couples closer together. A healthy and satisfying sex life is essential for a successful relationship. It can help partners to bond emotionally, communicate effectively, and feel more connected. When couples have a strong sexual connection, they are more likely to be happy and satisfied in their relationship.

Sex can also help to reduce stress and improve mood. During sex, the body releases endorphins, which are feel-good chemicals that can reduce anxiety and depression. A healthy sex life can also improve overall health, including reducing the risk of heart disease, boosting the immune system, and improving sleep quality.

How to Continue to Explore and Experiment in Your Sexual Relationship

Exploring and experimenting in your sexual relationship can help to keep things fresh and exciting. Communication is key when it comes to exploring new sexual experiences with your partner. Be open and honest about your desires and fantasies, and listen to your partner's wants and needs as well.

Trying new things in the bedroom can help to increase intimacy and build trust. You might try introducing sex toys or experimenting with different positions or techniques. You can also explore new fantasies or role-playing scenarios together. The key is to be respectful of each other's boundaries and to communicate throughout the process.

The Benefits of a Strong Sexual Connection with Your Partner

Having a strong sexual connection with your partner can have many benefits. It can improve emotional intimacy, communication, and overall relationship satisfaction. Couples who have a strong sexual connection are more likely to feel happy and fulfilled in their relationship.

Sex can also help to reduce stress and improve overall health. When you have regular sex, the body releases endorphins, which are feel-good chemicals that can reduce anxiety and depression. A healthy sex life can also improve sleep quality, boost the immune system, and reduce the risk of heart disease.

A healthy and satisfying sex life is an essential aspect of a successful relationship. It can improve emotional intimacy, communication, and overall relationship satisfaction. Exploring and experimenting in your sexual relationship can help to keep things fresh and exciting. The benefits of a strong sexual connection with your partner include reduced stress, improved mood, and better overall health. Communication is key when it comes to building a strong sexual connection with your partner. Be open and honest about your desires and needs, and be respectful of each other's boundaries. With effort and communication, you can build a strong and satisfying sexual relationship that enhances your overall relationship satisfaction.

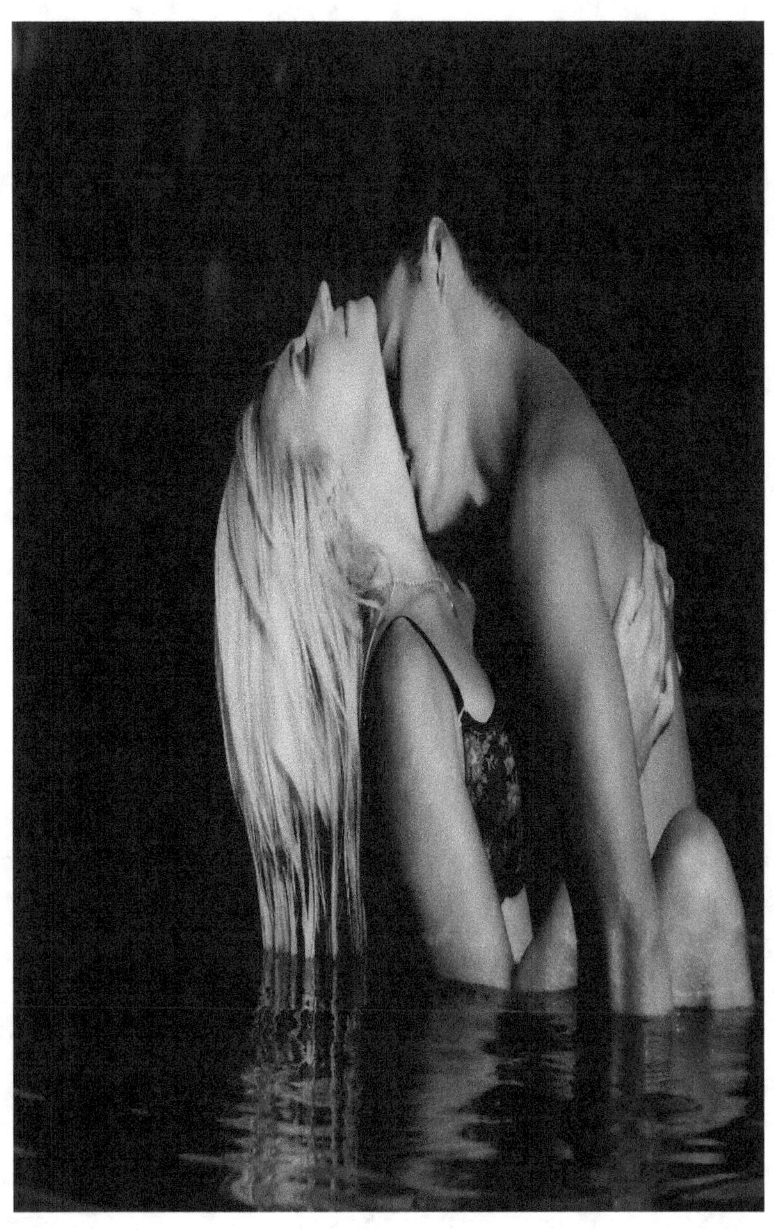

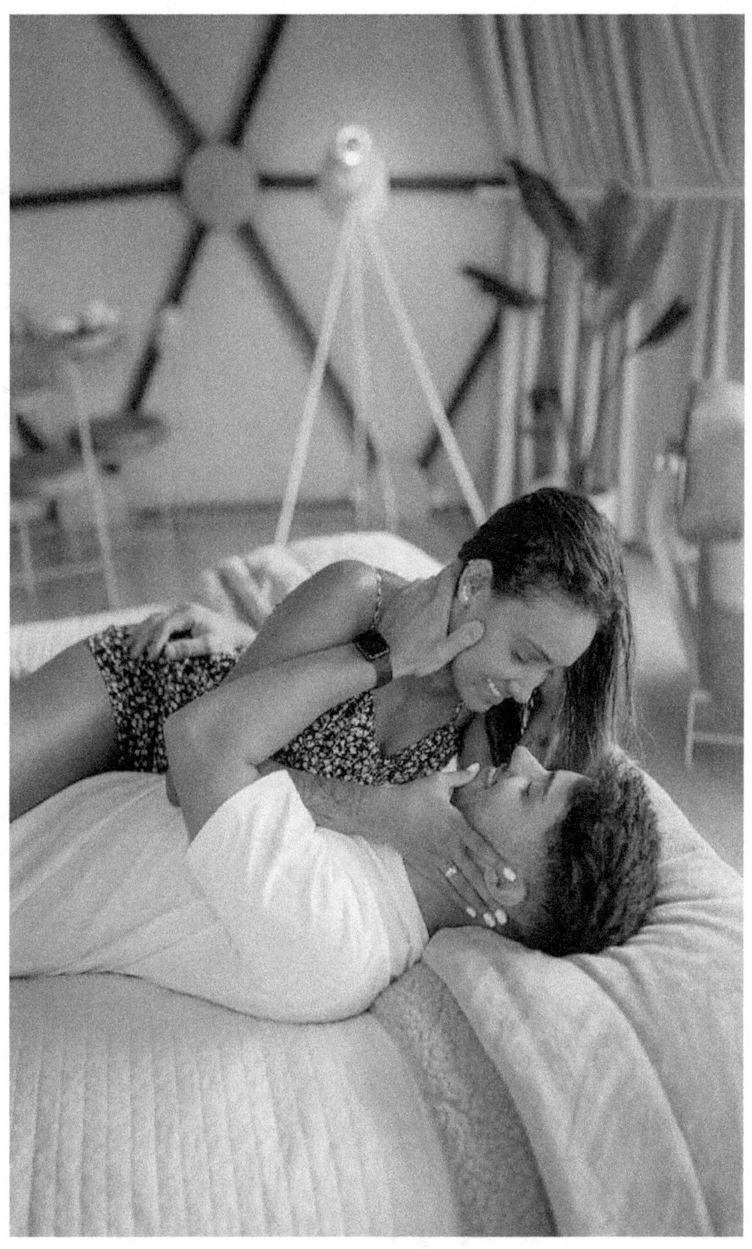